HORMONE BALANCING
THE BASICS

Focusing on the adrenals, the sex hormones and thyroid hormone

Leila Kirdani, MD

SECOND EDITION

4414 Culver Road
Rochester NY 14622
(585) 773-4777
www.drleila.com

Cover design by: Alaina Stark, AMS Marketing & Design, Inc.

Publishing Consult Mary K. Dougherty
Bootstrappublishing.net
And
Technical Coordinator and Book Promotional Manager
Barb Anderson
DMBookpro.com

Library of Congress Control Number: 2012948120
Paperback ISBN: 978-1481900492

First edition September 2012.
Second edition January 2013

Disclaimer: The information contained in this book is based upon the research and personal and professional experiences of the author. It is not intended as a substitute for consulting with your physician or other health care provider. The author is not responsible for any adverse effects of consequences resulting from the use of the suggestions or procedures discussed in this book. Should the reader have any questions concerning the appropriateness of any suggestions or procedures mentioned, the author strongly suggests consulting a professional healthcare advisor.
The names of the patients described in this book have been changed to protect their identities.

PRINTED IN THE USA

Dedication

To Dar: for being the rock that keeps me grounded

so I can fly to new heights.

Table of Contents

Introduction   7

Chapter 1
Why Am I So Tired? Balancing Adrenal Fatigue   13

Chapter 2
Hormone Balancing for Women: Why Am I So Miserable?   41

Chapter 3
Hormone Balancing for men: Why Am I So Miserable?   65

Chapter 4
Why am I so tired? Is my thyroid off?   84

Chapter 5
Conclusion & Recommended reading   97

Glossary of Terms   103

Acknowledgments

I would like to acknowledge Dr. Pamela Smith for creating the fellowship that gave me the knowledge I needed to truly make a difference in people's lives. I would also like to acknowledge Dr. Richard Moon for both the depth of his knowledge and his willingness to share it with me. Lastly I would like to acknowledge my family for their constant encouragement and support of my new ventures, and especially my children, Andrea and Neil for always being so proud of me.

Introduction

🍃 Patient Story

Lisa, a 47-year-old white female, felt like she was falling apart. She was irritable with her family and her employees. She had trouble both falling asleep and staying asleep, and her daytime energy levels were low. She had difficulty staying focused and felt that just getting through the day was overwhelming. Her periods were irregular—she was getting them every three to four months. She was having deep hot flashes that almost made her feel dizzy, especially in the morning. Lisa was very frustrated by the fact that while she exercised daily and ate well, she just couldn't get rid of the growing bulge around her middle.

Lisa told me that over the last few years her stress levels had increased. She and her husband owned a company that places temp workers, and with the downturn in the economy, the job pool had shrunk and they had to downsize their business. Lisa felt very responsible, and the stress of having to lay off people who had worked with them for a while was overwhelming.

After a complete work-up, I discovered that Lisa was suffering from adrenal fatigue, along with low levels of estrogen and progesterone. Lisa was started on a supplement regimen aimed at boosting her adrenals, along with bio-identical hormone replacement therapy. In two months Lisa felt back to her old self. Her energy was good, she was sleeping well, and she had lost six pounds. Her friends were commenting on how much better she looked. She couldn't believe the difference in how she felt.

Are you tired all the time? Worn out? Do you feel like you are not enjoying your life as much as you want to? Or perhaps you feel moody and irritable, and you snap at your loved ones?

If you can say yes to any of the above, this book was written for you. Many of us blame the way we feel on how busy our lives are. Sometimes we will go to our doctors with complaints of fatigue. The doctor may draw blood to look at our blood count and thyroid levels and tell us that everything looks "normal." He or she may tell us we are "just stressed" or maybe even a little depressed. However, the problem is not just that we are tired or have too much to do, or even that we are depressed. One of the most prevalent and important reasons why we feel miserable is that our hormones are out of balance. By balancing our hormones, we can balance our lives.

Hormones are essential to our happiness. Hormones help our cells function properly; when our hormone levels are low or out of balance, we can't feel good because none of our cells can work properly. This book is a simple guide to help you understand the basics of your hormones, how to recognize if your hormone levels are low or out of balance, and how to get them back into balance.

By hormones, I am referring to specifically cortisol, estrogen, progesterone, testosterone and the thyroid hormones T4, T3, and reverse T3. Cortisol is our "fight-or-flight" hormone. Because it regulates how our bodies react when we are under stress, cortisol is the most important hormone our body produces. Our body will shunt production of all of our other hormones into cortisol to keep us alive. If we don't balance cortisol, none of our other hormones will be balanced. Because most of us are under more stress than we were evolutionarily meant to be, cortisol issues are extremely prevalent in our society today.

Our sex hormones come next. We cannot experience joy, focus, or balance in life if our sex hormones are out of balance. Estrogen and progesterone for women and testosterone for men are an essential part of our well-being. They help us experience passion and creativity in all areas of our life.

The last hormone I will cover in this book is the group of hormones produced by the thyroid. The thyroid hormones regulate how hard all of our cells work and how much energy each cell produces. Because thyroid hormones are affected by all our other hormones, active thyroid hormone, or T3, is the hormone that I generally balance last. However, when the thyroid hormones are well-balanced, it is often the "icing on the cake" that makes us feel perfect.

I have come to know that hormones are the key to life. It is well-known among anti-aging doctors that we do not lose our hormones because we age; we age because we lose our hormones. If we understand that every single cell in our bodies has receptors for hormones and that hormones are an essential for all of our cells to function and to communicate, we can understand how this can be true. I know this book will help you on the way to your optimal health!

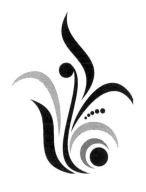

Chapter 1

Why Am I So Tired?
Balancing Adrenal Fatigue

Why Am I So Tired?

Do I Have Adrenal Fatigue?

Do you feel exhausted? Burned out? Do you crave sugar and caffeine? Do you get frequent cold and upper respiratory symptoms? Do you gain weight despite diet and exercise? Do you have muscle and joint pain? Do you feel irritable or anxious and less able to handle stress? You could be suffering from adrenal fatigue!

What Are the Adrenal Glands?

The adrenal glands are small, bean-sized glands which sit on top of each kidney. They are responsible for producing several hormones, including cortisol, aldosterone, DHEA, epinephrine, norepinephrine, and to a smaller extent testosterone, estrogen and progesterone. Cortisol has numerous functions in the body, including regulating electrolyte balance, blood pressure, inflammation, blood sugar, and brain function. Aldosterone is our main hormone of blood pressure regulation. DHEA, epinephrine and norepinephrine, as well as cortisol, all help us cope with stress.

What is Adrenal Fatigue?

Adrenal fatigue is a condition where the adrenal glands are unable to produce the amount of cortisol, or stress hormone, our bodies need to function during the day. Because of this dysfunction, there is not enough of this critical hormone to support our energy production or to help us cope with the stressors we experience. Adrenal fatigue can arise from either prolonged stress or after a shorter intense period of stress such as a surgery, a car accident, or even a divorce. Another cause of adrenal fatigue can be toxicity from heavy metals. Think of it this way: Our bodies were built for danger, not for chronic stress. We were designed to stay alive in the face of mortal danger. When the tiger jumps out of the bush at us, our cortisol (fight-or-flight hormone) immediately increases. This increase in cortisol produces changes in our body to help us stay alive in the face of danger. For example, increases in cortisol cause an increase in blood sugar so that our muscles and brain have fuel to run from the tiger. Part of our immune system is activated to produce inflammation so that if the tiger bites us, we can clot well and keep running. Another part of our immune system is suppressed; the natural killer cells which help us fight cancer, because we are not worried about cancer when we are facing a tiger. Additionally, blood flow to our intestines decreases because digesting and absorbing food is not a concern when we are faced with danger.

While these changes are important for our survival when faced with brief episodes of mortal danger, over long periods of time they can cause detrimental changes in the body. In the 21st century we are facing "tigers" all of the time. Our tigers today include childhood trauma, relationships, finances, time, job stress, car accidents, and a toxic environment, to name a few. Chronically increased blood sugar leads to belly fat and eventually diabetes. Chronically increased inflammation leads to numerous medical problems, including hypertension, asthma, allergies, arthritis, obesity, muscle and joint pain. With chronically suppressed natural killer cells, we have an increased risk of autoimmune diseases and cancer.

The adrenal glands were never designed to continually produce elevated levels of cortisol—we just weren't designed to be fighting a tiger twenty-four hours a day, seven days a week. After years of overproducing cortisol, the adrenal glands start to tire out, and then they can't produce enough cortisol to meet our daily needs. We all need some cortisol on a daily basis, especially in the morning.

Cortisol is one of the main "gases" in our "car's" tank. Cortisol affects the metabolism of every cell. Cortisol levels affect blood pressure, electrolyte balance—essentially how every cell functions. While our bodies always produce some cortisol to help us function, we should start producing more cortisol a few hours before we wake up. Because getting out of bed is one of the hardest things our bodies do, cortisol levels should peak in the morning. We have been lying flat all night, and suddenly we have to keep our blood pressure up to get blood to our brain, our muscles have to function, etc. A huge shift in metabolism happens the minute we get out of bed and put our feet on the floor, and it takes cortisol to make that happen. Ideally, cortisol levels should then taper over the course of the day and remain low but constant at night.

When our adrenal glands can no longer produce the amount of cortisol we need on a daily basis, we feel exhausted all the time. The cells that comprise our body can't function properly. Many of the changes that happen when our cortisol is too high also happen when our cortisol is too low. Think of it this way: Now we have fought the battle, acutely burning out our adrenal glands. We are lying on the battlefield, wounded, waiting for help to come. Our bodies shift to "survival mode."

When we are in survival mode, the goal of the body is to stay alive. That means the body increases blood sugar to keep fuel going to our heart, lungs, and brain. Inflammation is increased so we can clot any wounds that may have occurred during battle until help arrives. We are trying to conserve resources so blood flow to the intestines and kidneys is decreased. Natural killer cells are suppressed as well, because we are putting all of our resources into staying alive in the short term and not into fighting cancer and viruses. If we exist chronically in this state, we can suffer not only extreme fatigue, but any of the illnesses we see in our society today.

🍃 Patient Story

Linda, a 52-year-old yoga teacher, retired from a job in industry about five years ago and built her yoga studio. For the past two years, however, she has been suffering from progressive symptoms of arthritis. The pain in her joints and stiffness in her muscles had gotten to the point that she was unable to teach, and was in the process of applying for disability. Linda really did not like to take medicine, but she found herself taking an anti-inflammatory every night to be able to sleep. She just dealt with the pain during the day. Linda went to a rheumatologist who had diagnosed her with seronegative autoimmune arthritis, meaning it appeared that her body was attacking itself, yet none of the traditional tests for things like rheumatoid arthritis were positive.

Linda's saliva test showed that she was adrenal fatigued, and that her hormone levels were low. She was started on supplements, bio-identical hormone replacement therapy and a very low dose of cortisol. She could hardly believe the difference in her pain in just a few days. In a few weeks she was no longer taking the anti-inflammatory, and in a few months she was able to stop the cortisol and is being maintained on supplements and bio-identical hormone replacement therapy only.

Adrenal fatigue is the most common ailment I diagnose in my office. It is the reason why people are so tired. Most doctors do not look for adrenal fatigue. This syndrome of adrenal fatigue was first noticed in the 1800s. It was further delineated in the 1930s, when researchers began to understand more about the stress cycle. One very important finding by Hans Selye, the Canadian researcher who coined the term "stress," is that an organism actually responds to prolonged stress by decreased production of cortisol, and that the very worst stress is the perception of feeling trapped—by finances, jobs, and relationships, anything that makes us feel like we have lost control of our lives. Traditionally trained doctors are all schooled to be concerned about cortisol being too high, but rarely do they look for low cortisol levels.

There is a distinct bias in the medical community when it comes to adrenal fatigue. Doctors think that either your adrenal glands are working perfectly fine, or they have ceased to function—a condition known as "Addison's disease," which can land patients in the Intensive Care Unit. Part of this bias in the traditional medical community concerns the testing that is used for adrenal function. Standard testing for adrenal function done by traditionally trained doctors involves an ACTH test or adrenocorticotropin stimulation test. In this test a blood level of cortisol is drawn at baseline. The patient is then injected intravenously with adrenocorticotropin-stimulating hormone—the hormone produced by the pituitary gland to stimulate the adrenals to produce more cortisol when we are under stress. Repeat blood levels for cortisol are drawn, and if the cortisol level increases at all in the blood, the adrenals are thought to be functioning optimally.

The problem with this test is what it is really evaluating for is whether the adrenal glands can mount a "fight-flight" response. It actually tests only for how well the body responds to a tiger jumping out of the bush; it does not test how the adrenals are functioning on a day-to-day basis. The other problem with this test is that it is an "all-or-nothing" test, meaning that if the cortisol levels increases at all; your adrenals are considered normal. Clearly, however, if the cortisol level is supposed to go up 50 points and it only goes up 2 points, your adrenal function is definitely not optimal.

The other part of the bias that traditionally trained doctors have against looking for adrenal fatigue is the fact that often doctors are not the most healthy and well-balanced people. If we are not in touch with our own levels of stress, how can we help other people with theirs?

Consequences of Adrenal Fatigue

The consequences of adrenal fatigue are many. Fatigue is primary, along with the inability to cope with less significant stressors. Think about it—if your body can't produce more of the hormone that helps you deal with stress, every little stress will feel huge. This is why people feel more irritable, blow up at the kids inappropriately, or become tearful without good reason.

Increased blood sugar over time can lead to increased weight gain, especially around the abdomen, and eventually diabetes. Increased inflammation over time leads to all of the modern-day diseases, depending on where your genetic "weak link" is. This can range from autoimmune disorders and thyroid problems to cardiovascular disease and intestinal issues. Consider how many problems are caused by inflammation—arthritis, asthma, high blood pressure, muscle aches and joint pain. The suppression of natural killer cells by low cortisol increases our risk for cancer and infections. Decreased blood flow to the gut causes constipation, diarrhea, irritable bowel, and in general decreased absorption of nutrients. It can feel like we are breaking down.

It is extremely common for people with adrenal fatigue to feel exhausted during the day and yet have difficulty getting to sleep at night. There is a very close link between low cortisol levels during the day and higher levels at night. Often people with adrenal fatigue feel like they get their "second wind" around 9:00 at night, and then try to make up for everything they feel like they did not get done during the day. It is also very common for people with adrenal fatigue to wake up between 1:00 and 3:00 in the morning. This is typically the time when the body has run out of its last food stores, cortisol levels are at an all-time low for the day, and the body senses that the energy supply to the brain and other vital organs is dangerously low. We are designed to survive. Our brain will actually wake us up in emergency mode so that our bodies will make more cortisol to keep us alive. People usually experience this as waking up and not being able to "shut off" their heads.

An added consequence to low cortisol levels is that the body will steal other hormones to make cortisol. For example, if we are struggling to produce cortisol, our bodies will "steal" progesterone and turn it into cortisol. This puts the body into a low progesterone state, which can lead to irritability, anxiety, insomnia, and panic. In addition, for women in particular, this can lead to weight gain in the hips and thighs, palpitations, severe premenstrual syndrome, and an increased risk of breast cancer.

Patient Story

Cathy, a 46-year-old white female, presented with complaints that she just wasn't feeling like herself. She had terrible swings in energy and anxiety during different times of the month. With ovulation and when her period came, she would feel exhausted, and then other times she would feel absolutely wired. She had gone to her OB-GYN thinking that her problem was related to sex hormones, but they only offered her an antidepressant. She was not a complainer, but when asked, she said she felt so tired that even cooking dinner for her family felt like an absolute chore. She wanted to be a good mom and enjoy her kids, but mostly she felt bothered by them. Cathy was embarrassed by her difficulty in comprehending her children's homework. She felt foggy and had difficulty remembering words.

When I looked at Cathy's adrenal function, she was virtually flat-lined. There was no increase in cortisol in the morning and her levels were well below optimal functioning all day long, except at night when she had trouble staying asleep. I started Cathy on supplements to support her adrenals and a lot of 7-keto DHEA. She started feeling better within weeks. She couldn't believe it wasn't her sex hormones, but when she educated herself about adrenal fatigue, she realized that her life of perfectionism and always pushing herself to do more had really worn her out.

How Do I Know if I Have Adrenal Fatigue?

If you are experiencing any of the symptoms above, including chronic fatigue, irritability, tearfulness, muscle and joint pain, craving sweets and caffeine, frequent colds and upper respiratory infections, or lack of enjoyment of life, then you may be suffering from adrenal fatigue. (I have included a brief symptom list at the end of this chapter.) Stressors that contribute to adrenal fatigue include divorce, car accidents, surgery, single parenting, childhood trauma, abusive relationships, perfectionism, and a toxic environment.

The best way to test for adrenal fatigue is through salivary testing. Testing for hormones through saliva is more accurate than blood testing for a few reasons. The first is that merely getting a needle-stick to obtain a blood sample is painful and can raise your cortisol levels. Another reason is that blood levels of hormones do not accurately reflect the levels of hormones inside of cells. We are only as healthy as our cells. In blood, hormones are present in three different ways. They can be found free (unbound) and are available to be taken up by the cells to use for metabolism, which is the aspect we want to know about.

Hormones also come bound to huge carrier proteins which cannot cross the cell membrane—this portion is not able to be used by the cells. Lastly, they can be loosely bound to albumin. This portion can go into either the free or bound pools, depending on what the body needs. Because saliva glands excrete their contents, more of what is on the inside of the cell ends up in the saliva. Additionally, saliva does not have carrier proteins. Obtaining four saliva samples over the course of the day allows us to determine exactly where the adrenals are throughout the day. A twenty-four hour urine collection for cortisol can also show if the cortisol production for the day is too low; however, it cannot tell us where the low points and high points may be.

Treatment for Adrenal Fatigue

The treatment of adrenal fatigue requires a multifactorial approach. The basic tenets include lifestyle changes like diet, nutrition, finding ways to de-stress, supplementation, and detoxification.

Patients often ask me, "How long will it take?" The answer to that question depends on the severity of the adrenal fatigue to begin with, and how well the patient takes care of his/herself. Quite honestly, the people who invest in lifestyle changes the most are often the people who get well the quickest.

The other big factor in turning adrenal fatigue around is changing the stresses in our lives. I have many women who are perfectionists and drive themselves to achieve constantly. Because they are unable to change and learn to relax a little, they are constantly on the brink and slipping back into adrenal fatigue.

Diet and Nutrition: Making sure the body gets enough protein is one of the most important things that can be done for adrenal fatigue. Protein helps every single aspect of the body—not just making hormones, but healthy brain function, immune system function, energy levels, and obviously muscle health. I cannot emphasize this enough. Taking in adequate amounts of protein can make a significant change in energy levels.

What is enough? For people who have adrenal fatigue, I recommend one and a half grams of protein per kilograms of body weight per day. For example, a 70-kilogram person would need to eat 105 grams of protein per day. If you exercise more than three hours a week, you may need to take in two grams of protein per kilogram of body weight per day.

The more nutrients we can feed our bodies, the better it is, and so eating lots of vegetables every day is important. Among anti-aging doctors the current recommendation is 10-15 servings of fruits and vegetables a day! To achieve this level of intake, juicing can be quite helpful. While fruit is good for us, it can raise blood sugars slightly, and should always be eaten with some kind of protein.

While we often crave sugar and caffeine when our cortisol is low, these items make adrenal fatigue worse! As much as possible, avoid processed foods with additives and preservatives—chemicals increase stress on the body. Not only is processed food lacking in nutrients, the body often uses up more nutrients to break down than it actually replaces.

Avoiding common food allergens such as dairy products, wheat, corn, shellfish, and peanuts is beneficial for your entire body. Food allergies create inflammation, which can perpetuate adrenal fatigue. If you know your blood type, you can follow Peter D'Adamo's *Eat Right 4 Your Type* diet plans. If you stick to eating mostly the foods that are either beneficial or neutral for your blood type, you are more likely to be more efficiently breaking down and absorbing the food you eat. Hunger is also very stressful to our bodies, so eating small meals every three hours will help the adrenals heal.

Supplements: Replacing electrolytes is very important for the treatment of adrenal fatigue. Electrolytes drive every intra-cellular process we have—from taking in nutrients, to clearing out wastes, to making the very molecules our cells use for energy called ATP (adenosine triphosphate).

People with adrenal fatigue tend to be lower in sodium than potassium, so replacing at a one-to-one ratio of sodium and potassium is best. In my practice I recommend alfalfa, a "green" that raises sodium and potassium equally. Another way to do this is with sea salt. Sea salt also has that one-to-one ratio of sodium to potassium, as opposed to table salt, which has no potassium whatsoever and therefore puts our bodies out of balance. In his book *Adrenal Fatigue: The 21st Century Syndrome,* James Wilson recommends trying one-quarter teaspoon of sea salt in eight ounces of water. If the water tastes better (not salty), he recommends continuing to add quarter-teaspoons until the water does taste salty, backing off by one quarter teaspoon, and drinking this mix twice daily. I find many people do not tolerate sea salt orally, and so find the water too salty from the get-go. Another way to utilize sea salt is sea-salt baths. Place one-quarter cup of sea salt in bathwater and soak for ten-fifteen minutes. The skin will absorb the electrolytes from the sea salt.

Getting enough B vitamins is also quite essential. B vitamins are needed by so many intracellular processes, and we just don't get enough from our diets. A good B-100 complex is a great place to start, but it is important to add extra B12, as most B complexes do not include enough B12. Optimum doses of vitamin B12 are typically 2000 micrograms per day. Minerals are found in high quantities in the adrenal glands, so a good multi-mineral supplement is essential. Adrenal glandular supplements are extremely helpful, as they have all the nutrients adrenal glands need, in addition to providing energetic support needed by the adrenal glands.

Aside from these basics to help the adrenals function better, probably the most crucial nutrient to heal adrenal fatigue is DHEA (dihydroepiandrosterone). DHEA is our "stress reserve tank." It is the main precursor hormone to cortisol. DHEA helps us with energy, mood, how quickly we think, muscle and bone health, gut health, and immunity. The adrenals actually want to produce fifteen times more DHEA than cortisol. It is as if they want their reserve tank full and to have those energy reserves spill over into cortisol. Under stress, the body uses up DHEA. The body makes less as we age, so supplementation is essential. Men can replace DHEA at doses of 50-100 milligrams per day in the morning. Women, however, need to use a metabolite of DHEA called 7-keto DHEA. The problem with regular DHEA is that it can convert to other hormones like testosterone and estrogen in women's bodies, causing side effects in doses above 25 milligrams. These include acne, facial hair, headaches, and increased blood pressure. 7-keto DHEA stays as DHEA in the body, so it just fills up that reserve tank nicely. Women should start at 100-200 milligrams of 7-keto DHEA per day, again in the morning. How much you need depends on how much you are using up every day, so how much stress you are under. This can include psychological stress, physical stress, and what I call "internal stress," meaning people who have a lot of internal inflammation.

If we understand that psychological stress is one of our biggest sources of stress, it is easy to see how important supplements are that will help to mitigate those stressors. Supplements that help us with stress include L-theanine, an amino acid which helps to keep us calm and focused without being sedating. I recommend L-theanine for those who have a lot of "internal angst"—they worry a lot about everything. A dose of 200 milligrams twice daily is a good initial dose.

Niacinamide is a form of niacin, or vitamin B3, that balances brain waves, so it helps cut the chatter in our heads. When we are stressed, we often keep thinking the same thoughts over and over, and this keeps our stress going. Niacinamide helps to stop our overthinking. It improves focus and can help with sleep. For many people, 250 milligrams twice daily is helpful.

For the people who are "wound up" at night or who are still trying to fight that tiger despite the fact that they are exhausted, rhodiola can be quite helpful. Rhodiola is an herb that helps to lower elevated cortisol levels over time. Even though a patient's cortisol level may be low, they can still be "wired," meaning they are still in the mode where they are trying to fight a tiger and demanding their bodies produce more cortisol. This state is in part what wore them out to begin with, and to help break that chronic fight/flight, rhodiola at 250 milligrams twice a day can go a long way.

Finally, Relora is a blend of herbs that acts as what we call an adrenal gland "adaptogen"—meaning it supports the adrenals if they are running low and calms them down if they are on overdrive. 75-150 milligrams twice a day can help us cope with the feeling that "our world is too busy."

Detoxify: Remember that I mentioned that toxicity from heavy metals is a major cause of adrenal fatigue? Well, in order to heal our adrenal glands, we need to detoxify. Heavy metals are metals that should not be found in large amounts in our environment, but due to industrialization, they are more present than they ought to be. We have all heard about lead, but mercury is the EPA's number one toxin. Mercury is found in industrial waste, vaccines, and metal dental fillings. Cadmium is in cigarette smoke and petroleum products, so gasoline fumes and many of our lotions and shampoos contain cadmium. Arsenic is in industrial waste and pressure-treated wood, so it gets into groundwater. Aluminum is also in industrial waste, canned goods, vaccines, powders as an anti-clumping agent, and cosmetics.

As you can see, heavy metals are ubiquitous! Fortunately, we can detoxify with blue-green algae, like chlorella, which bind heavy metals in our intestines and carry them out of our bodies. I have also had good results with heavy metal foot-pads, which feel like "voodoo," but actually do work to ironically pull metals out through the lymph tissue. You wake up, and the pad you have worn is full of metals!

Lifestyle Changes: This is about balance!.Lifestyle changes are essential to help our adrenal glands heal. What are your stressors? How can you deal with them differently? Can you find more time to be by yourself? What do you enjoy doing the most? What "fills you up"? Try not to do any work for an hour before bed to help relax your mind. Don't forget the importance of regular exercise, and get enough sleep! This means 8-9 hours a night.

Relaxation Exercises: As we work to change the stressors in our lives, there are a few quick ways to "de-stress." Deep breathing can go a long way to help us let go of stress and tension. Five times a day, get to a place where you are alone and take three deep breaths. Breathe in through your nose and out through your mouth. As you exhale, consciously feel your body relaxing, the stress and tension leaving your muscles. An expanded version of this exercise can be done before bed. Sit in a comfortable position and take your three deep breaths. Feel your body relaxing, but start from your head and go down to your toes. First, feel your neck and shoulders relax, next breath your arms, back, stomach, and third breathe your legs and feet. Stay in this position for another 30 seconds, holding on to your relaxed state. Doing this exercise before bed actually helps our bodies and minds relax, allowing us to heal more deeply overnight.

How else can you relax? Meditation is extremely effective. Other modalities such as massage therapy, acupuncture, aromatherapy and energy work can be very helpful to the adrenal glands.

Healing your adrenals can be as easy as removing what shouldn't be in your body (toxins) and replacing what should be in your body (good nutrients). Like your grandmother used to say, eat right, get plenty of rest, and exercise!

Symptom List for Adrenal Fatigue

- Fatigue, often extreme exhaustion that does not improve with sleep
- Difficulty getting up in the morning
- Craving carbohydrates, sugar, caffeine, and salty foods
- Symptoms worsen when meals are skipped
- Poor libido
- Decreased ability to cope with stress
- Difficulty concentrating and maintaining focus
- Worsening memory
- Increased irritability, moodiness and anxiety
- Lack of enjoyment with life
- More frequent illnesses, especially upper respiratory illnesses
- Difficulty recovering from illnesses
- Worsening symptoms of PMS
- Light-headedness or dizziness when standing up quickly or getting out of bed

- Poor productivity at work

- Energy low in the afternoon, while energy improves (second wind) at night

- Mid-thoracic back pain, heartburn, or sinus pressure

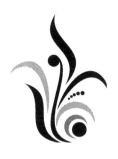

Chapter 2

Hormone Balancing for Women

Why Am I So Miserable?

Hormone Balancing For Women:

Why Am I So Miserable?

Do you have trouble sleeping? Are you irritable and moody? Are you gaining weight even though your diet and activity haven't changed? Have you lost your passion for life? Do you just want to feel like yourself again? You could be suffering from hormonal imbalance!

🌱 Patient Story

Lilly, a 52-year-old white female, felt much older. Ever since menopause she was moody and irritable, and worst of all was the painful vaginal dryness she had developed. She felt like her life was over.

Following her studies, I started Lilly on some adrenal support, but mostly high levels of estrogen and progesterone. Within six months she was back to feeling like herself again. Her mood had improved significantly and her vaginal dryness completely resolved.

What Are Hormones?

Hormones are substances produced in special organs in the body, such as the ovaries, testicles, and thyroid, and then released into the bloodstream. They then travel to cells in other parts of the body where the hormone then exerts its characteristic effect. Our human hormones include estrogen, testosterone, progesterone, cortisol, thyroid, DHEA and, believe it or not, vitamin D.

Why Is This Significant?

Hormones are responsible for the vital functioning of our bodies. Remember that every single cell in our bodies has receptors for hormones, so no cell can function well without the appropriate amount of hormone. We tend to think of sex hormones in terms of our secondary sex characteristics and libido, but in fact estrogen has over 400 functions in a woman's body, and testosterone has the same for men. Let's start from the top and work our way down with the functions that first estrogen and then progesterone have in a woman's body.

In the brain estrogen is responsible for helping us to make serotonin, which is our neurotransmitter of joy. Without enough estrogen we just don't feel happy, and can even suffer from depression. Estrogen also helps with short-term memory and word recall, to which many postmenopausal women can relate, as we have all struggled to think of a name or word.

Estrogen is extremely important for the cardiovascular system on many levels. Estrogen, when well-balanced with progesterone, decreases clot formation and actually thins the blood. This is completely opposite to what pharmaceutical estrogens do in the body. Pharmaceutical estrogens, because they are different molecules than our own natural estrogens, have been shown to increase the risk of heart attacks and strokes. I will discuss these differences in greater depth in future sections. Estrogen decreases blood pressure and reduces plaque formation, as well as increasing good cholesterol (HDL) and lowering bad cholesterol (LDL). Most importantly, for both heart health and overall body health, estrogen, again when well-balanced with progesterone, is a woman's most powerful anti-inflammatory, so it can prevent the basic process of increased inflammation that contributes to heart disease and all other diseases.

Like all other cells, the cells that line our intestines need estrogen for their healthy metabolism, so when we are low in estrogen, we can suffer from symptoms like constipation, irritable bowel, and heartburn. Since estrogen helps insulin to be more effective, when our estrogen is low, we are at greater risk for diabetes, as our bodies will not process food as well.

Most of us are aware of estrogen's important role in the prevention of bone loss—a great concern for postmenopausal women. Estrogen is responsible for preventing the breakdown of bone, so low estrogen levels, among other things, can lead to osteoporosis.

Estrogen has many other functions in the body, including helping with collagen formation and therefore improving elasticity of the skin. Estrogen helps skin cells retain water, so when we are low in estrogen, our skin, hair, and nails all seem dry and saggy.

🍂 Patient Story

Sandra came to me with the complaint of peri-menopausal symptoms. She was irritable and had problems sleeping. She was tired all of the time and had no libido. Sandra complained that her skin was dry and saggy. She was gaining weight, but felt too tired to go to the gym.

I performed salivary testing for cortisol and sex hormones. All of Sandra's levels were low. I started her on adrenal support as well as bioidentical hormone replacement. At first Sandra didn't feel much difference, but once I raised her hormone levels, she felt great. She had energy and was back at the gym. Her sleep improved and she felt 10 years younger.

What about progesterone? Like estrogen, progesterone has numerous important functions in our bodies, but probably the most important function it has is that it balances our estrogen. Strong estrogens like estradiol and estrone can cause growth—growth of the uterine lining which is shed monthly with our menstrual cycles, growth of breast buds through menarche, and potentially the growth of breast and uterine cancers. Natural progesterone, unlike synthetic progestins, actually decreases this powerful effect of estrogen. Progesterone decreases estradiol production, increases its breakdown, and down-regulates the growth-promoting "alpha" estrogen receptors in breast and uterine tissue. Studies of women who had lower levels of progesterone over the course of their lifetimes had increased incidence of both breast and uterine cancers.

In the brain, progesterone stimulates the production of our neurotransmitter GABA, or gamma-aminobutyric acid, which is the neurotransmitter that helps us feel like "everything is okay in life." Without enough progesterone, we can be more anxious and irritable. Low progesterone levels relative to estrogen levels near the end of our menstrual cycle is primarily what causes the irritability and mood swings that go along with premenstrual syndrome. Progesterone also helps to quicken the speed of thinking, as well as promoting healthy sleep patterns. With regard to the heart, progesterone exerts a positive effect in many ways. It is the balance of estrogen and progesterone that decreases inflammation. If we are low in progesterone relative to our estrogen, increased inflammation and an increased risk of blood clots can occur. Progesterone is in part responsible for fluid and electrolyte balance, as well as relaxing artery walls, so it helps maintain healthy blood pressure levels.

Progesterone helps us to metabolize carbohydrates, so when our progesterone is low, we have that feeling that we can just look at a carbohydrate and gain weight! Progesterone also helps with the internal strength of bone.

🍃 Patient Story

Laurel was very health-conscious. She ate a mostly organic diet, worked out daily, and was overall very active. She had trouble understanding, then, why for the last few years she had become increasingly impatient and irritable. Her PMS had become increasingly worse. Laurel felt awful about snapping at her children during these times.

I found that Laurel's progesterone levels were very low during the second half of her cycle. By replacing her progesterone with natural progesterone cream, Laurel's irritability and PMS completely resolved. Now Laurel recognizes that in more stressful months she needs to use more progesterone, and in less stressful months she can use less.

I would like to spend a little time on testosterone for women. We are incorrectly biased in our society, thinking that testosterone is the hormone that increases libido for both men and women. Testosterone's role in libido for men goes without question; however, for women it is a little more complex. For women, there is no one single hormone that creates sex drive. When you think about it, the roles of men and women in sustaining the species are fairly different. While a man's role is to propagate the species, the women's role is to protect their young. Women's bodies are set up so that we have lower libido and are even less fertile at times of stress. For a healthy libido in women, we need to have all of our hormones in place and balanced—not just testosterone.

Testosterone does have other important functions in a woman's body, however, including increasing muscle and bone strength, and helping with our self-confidence, focus, motivation, and drive.

It's All About Balance!

I can't emphasize enough that it is the balance between estrogen and progesterone that most helps with our health. Health problems can occur and symptoms can appear if the balance between these hormones is off in either direction. Estrogen dominance, or having too much estrogen relative to our progesterone, is the most common form of imbalance that I see. This happens because of stress and the toxicity of the environment.

We have discussed in the adrenal chapter that when we are stressed, our bodies will "steal" progesterone to turn it into cortisol. Evolutionarily, it made sense that if the tribe was at war or if the tribe was starving, it was not the time to be making babies, so our bodies took the hormone we needed for fertility (progesterone) and turned it into the hormone we needed for survival. In our twenty-first century we may not be warring or starving, but we are suffering more constant psychological stressors.

With regards to toxicity, we are exposed to both xenoestrogens and heavy metals. Xenoestrogens are chemicals in our environment that mimic estrogen in the body. They are found in solvents, insecticides, and pesticides, and put the body into a state of being constantly estrogen-dominant. Heavy metals were discussed in the adrenal chapter. They adversely affect the ability of the body to produce adequate amounts of hormones.

When we are estrogen-dominant, we can experience problems with anxiety, panic, palpitations, insomnia, heavy menstrual cycles, weight gain in the hips, thighs, and tummy, and an increased risk of fibroids, endometriosis, and breast and uterine cancers. We can also experience increased inflammation—so, muscle and joint aches, along with an increased risk for heart attacks and strokes.

On the other hand, too much progesterone rarely occurs, and when it does, it is usually a result of over-replacement. The most common symptom seen when there is too much progesterone is fatigue, but this imbalance can also cause bloating, swelling of the extremities, constipation, hot flashes, and bladder leakage. Too much progesterone, or not enough estrogen, can also cause depression, insomnia, and vaginal dryness.

It is easy to see why many women don't feel as good as they can after they go through menopause. Fortunately, there is a solution! It comes in the form of bio-identical hormone replacement therapy (BHRT). Because of the influences of the media and traditional medicine, many women are concerned with the inherent "dangers" of BHRT. I will address the most common concern in the next section.

🍃 Patient Story

Linda was strongly encouraged to come and see me by her therapist because of her depression. She was often teary and had difficulty handling regular life situations. Her mood was so low so much of the time that she often felt like ending her life. Linda knew her low mood was probably related to her low estrogen levels since menopause, but she was convinced that estrogen replacement therapy would mean she would get breast cancer. She had a strong family history of breast cancer and was well-read on the effects of traditional hormone replacement therapy and the increased risk of breast cancer.

After much education on the differences between traditional hormone replacement therapy and bio-identical hormone replacement therapy, Linda was convinced to try BHRT. The difference for Linda was unbelievable. Her depression lifted and she felt like she had a new lease on life.

I Heard Hormones Were Bad For You— Can Estrogen Cause Cancer?

This question initiates the discussion of bio-identical hormones versus traditional hormone replacement therapy (HRT). Bio-identical hormones are hormones made from plants to be the exact same molecule our bodies naturally produce. Because they are identical in structure to a naturally occurring molecule, bioidentical hormones are not able to be patented. Traditional HRT uses hormones that are not the same molecule. Pharmaceutical companies alter the original molecule because they cannot "own" a naturally occurring molecule. Our bodies are very complex and need the exact key to fit our molecular "locks," or receptor sites on cells. If you think small changes in structure don't matter, look at the difference between estradiol and testosterone.

Just a few chemical bonds and a few hydrogen atoms comprise the entire molecular difference between men and women!

Estradiol   **Testosterone**

For many years, the most commonly prescribed form of HRT for women was Premarin. Premarin, or conjugated equine estrogen, is derived from pregnant horse urine, and contains over 27 different estrogen compounds that are molecularly different from human estrogens. Our bodies can only use two of these compounds, and then need to break down the other 25 which are not usable. Most of these estrogens are broken down by metabolic pathways that generate carcinogenic intermediaries.

Side effects of synthetic estrogens including Premarin include: breast tenderness, high blood pressure, vaginal bleeding, gallstones, blood clots, headaches, leg cramps, insulin resistance, worsening of uterine fibroids and endometriosis, jaundice, and even cancer. Premarin has been shown to cause DNA damage, and therefore increases the risk of breast and uterine cancers.

The most commonly prescribed progestin in the United States was Provera, or medroxyprogestin acetate. The difference in structure between natural progesterone and Provera can be seen below.

Natural Progesterone   **Provera**

Because of these two little side chains of difference, progestins act very differently from progesterone in the body. Some of the side effects of progestins include: increasing the formation of clots and plaques, promoting insulin resistance, significantly lowering HDL, and increasing LDL. Unlike our own natural progesterone, which we need for a healthy pregnancy, progestins are contraindicated in pregnancy due to causing birth defects. Provera has been shown to cause cancer.

What significantly changed all this were the findings of The Women's Health Initiative. This study, which included over 150,000 women, showed that women taking Premarin and Provera together had an increased risk of cancer, blood clots, and heart disease. When this study was published, millions of women stopped taking their HRT, and sales of synthetic hormones dropped by over $1 billion annually!.Unfortunately, a lot of confusion was generated on the part of the pharmaceutical companies so that doctors and patients began to think all estrogens were bad. This is definitely not the case. More recent evidence has shown that bio-identical hormones, when used in the correct balance, actually prevent cancer!

🍃 Patient Story

Kate had a history of breast cancer. Both she and her traditional doctors felt that her breast cancer was a result of her being on

Premarin for over 20 years. When she came to me, she was tired and achy—all of her joints hurt, and she had already had surgery on her thumb and wrist for arthritis. Because she had adrenal fatigue, I opted to address her adrenal issues first; however, her inflammation did not completely resolve. After a lengthy discussion on the pros and cons of replacement therapy, Kate chose to go on BHRT. While not a night-and-day difference, Kate has noticed that her energy has improved significantly and her inflammation is much less.

If We Use Bio-Identical Hormones, We Aren't Aging "Naturally"

This is the second most common question I am asked, and here is my answer: First of all, it is only in the last 100 years that we have lived past middle age—humans used to die in our 50s. In fact, getting rid of our hormones is often nature's way of getting rid of us! Now that we are living into our 70s and 80s, we are seeing the effects of living without hormones—the likelihood of all disease is increased. The rates of diabetes, heart disease, high cholesterol, arthritis, and cancer all increase as we age. Secondly, we are all living more stressful, toxic lives than we were evolutionarily made for, so we are definitely not aging "naturally" to begin with.

Sign Me Up! I Want to Feel Great! Where Do I Start?

It is important to start with lifestyle changes to help balance hormones because of the effects of stress and diet on hormonal dysregulation. It means getting back to the basics again—eating good food, getting enough rest, and regular exercise. Not only will improving diet and lifestyle help us to feel better even if we do not choose to use hormone replacement, but it will help our hormones to work better if we do choose to replace them. Let us cover all of these aspects in a little more depth.

Diet and Nutrition: As we discussed in the adrenal chapter, eating plenty of fresh fruits and vegetables is important to hormone balancing. Brassica vegetables in particular, such as broccoli, cauliflower and Brussels sprouts, contain a compound called indole-3-carbinol, which promotes healthy estrogen metabolism, thus helping to prevent breast cancer. Avoiding processed foods which are nutrient-deficient, such as junk food and soda, as well as limiting caffeine and sugar, is also important. Getting enough protein is also very helpful for hormone balancing. Eating that one and a half grams per kilogram of body weight of protein per day helps your body produce healthy amounts of hormones.

I would like to make a special comment on soy products. In recent years there has been a growing controversy about soy. This comes from misunderstanding about the role of phytoestrogens. Phytoestrogens are very different from xenoestrogens in how they affect the body. Whereas xenoestrogens stimulate estrogen growth receptors and cause estrogen dominance, phytoestrogens act to block those estrogen growth receptors so we get the positive effects of estrogen without all the harmful effects. There is also growing awareness that soy can be unhealthy for the thyroid. This is because soy inhibits thyroid hormone production.

To make any significant alterations, however, one would need to eat 50-60 grams of soy per day, which most Americans don't even come close to consuming. At quantities less than this, I am in favor of soy for most people.

Getting Enough Rest: Remember, this is about balance! Stress uses up our hormones and we turn sex hormones into cortisol for survival. We absolutely have to work on adrenal issues if we are working to balance our hormones. This includes getting adequate sleep, having "play" time, and detoxifying heavy metals!

Exercise: Exercise has actually been shown to help with hormone balance because it decreases the amount of testosterone that converts to estrogen, which helps balance estrogen levels. Exercise also helps adrenal issues, which significantly bolster hormone balancing by helping progesterone stay as progesterone.

Supplements: To balance our sex hormones, we need to build on the base of healthy adrenals, so many of the supplement recommendations are the same, starting with B vitamins and electrolytes. A good B-100 complex is a great place to start, but it is important to add extra B12, as most B complexes do not include enough B12. Also, replacing electrolytes with an electrolyte drink (watch the sugar!), sea salt in water, or alfalfa is crucial to healthy body function and hormone balance. Omega-3 fatty acids help to balance hormones, because healthy fats are needed for hormone production. Most people should take 1000 milligrams of omega-3 fatty acids per day.

There are herbs that help balance hormones as well. My favorite is chasteberry, because it works to balance estrogen, progesterone, and cortisol. Most of us need all three areas addressed. Black cohosh and dong quai help to increase estrogen levels, but it is usually low progesterone and cortisol issues that are the cause of imbalance, not high estrogen.

Beyond the Basics – BHRT

For many women, however, these measures are just not enough. Fortunately, there is bio-identical hormone replacement therapy. By using BHRT we work to bring the body back in balance by imitating the body's natural processes as much as possible. Hormones are replaced to the extent that the symptoms caused by the natural decrease in production of hormones are alleviated. Of course, it is best to find a provider who is trained in the use of bio-identical hormones. Providers who are trained in the use of BHRT most often prescribe BHRT in the form of creams that are applied to the skin. Creams mimic the body's natural processes more than pills do because, for the most part, the gut was not designed to take in hormones. Additionally, estrogen and testosterone taken by mouth can increase inflammation in the liver when broken down in the gut. Hormone creams are made by compounding pharmacies. Compounding pharmacies harken back to the days when pharmacists actually made things up just for you. To ensure you are getting a quality product, look for accreditation through the Pharmacy Compounding Accreditation Board (PCAB), because you know they will have quality products.

While many women who start on a program of supplementation and BHRT feel better within a few months, it can take up to a year to achieve optimal health. It is extremely important to educate yourself as to the various options out there. Read reference books and articles.

Listen to your body. Document changes you are experiencing, and talk with your health professionals. Remember—optimal health is always achievable!

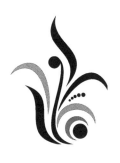

Chapter 3

Hormone Balancing for Men

Hormone Replacement for Men:

Why Am I So Miserable?

Why am I so grouchy? My wife and kids don't want to be around me! Why do my joints ache? I can't remember things as well as I used to, and I feel clumsy. I've got a pot belly and I just want to sit on the couch and be left alone. It can't be my testosterone level—if it were, I would have erectile dysfunction!

🌿 Patient Story

Justin, an amateur cyclist, came to me because he wanted to improve his performance. Other men that he bicycled with were on testosterone replacement and were able to outride him. He felt that his mood was fine, and that he was dealing adequately with stress.

After testing, I discovered that Justin's testosterone levels were only slightly low; however, he was suffering from some adrenal fatigue. While supporting his adrenals, I also opted to replace testosterone. Justin told me at his next visit that he couldn't believe how much better he felt. He really hadn't realized how miserable he was now that he felt better. And, of course, his cycling improved as well!

I Know I've Got Enough Testosterone!

How do you know? It is true that men do not go through "menopause" like women, but men do go through andropause. Andropause is the gradual decline in testosterone levels as men age. This decline occurs more slowly than the hormonal decline seen in women—over decades rather than just years—so men may not notice, as women do, the changes that occur with this decline.

What happens when testosterone levels drop? We tend to think that as long as a man can still achieve an erection, his testosterone level must be okay, but this is just not true. As testosterone levels decline, every cell that has a receptor for testosterone will not function as well. Basically that means every cell in the body! Aside from the genitals, the brain and the heart have the most testosterone receptors, so these organs suffer the most when testosterone levels drop.

Symptoms of Andropause

- Loss of drive and competitive edge
- Stiffness and pain in muscles and joints
- Falling level of fitness
- Decreased effectiveness of workouts
- Fatigue
- Depression/Low Mood
- Irritability
- Osteoporosis
- Anemia
- And then finally, reduced libido and potency

🍃 Patient Story

Jake was a partner in a busy architectural firm and had just turned 60. While he was able to keep up at work, he felt like he was losing his "edge." He had already been to an anti-aging physician who had started him on testosterone cream, but was unwilling to push his dose above 100 milligrams.

Jake's salivary testing showed that he was adrenal-fatigued and his testosterone level was still low. I explained to Jake how his body was stealing testosterone to convert it into cortisol. We opted to place him on adrenal support and increase his testosterone. Jake now feels great—he is sixty and keeping up with thirty-year-olds. He states that he can now do anything he wants, including boating, working out, and keeping up with his job demands.

Andropause is a Killer!

Aside from being the cause of the "grouchy couch potato," low testosterone levels actually have serious implications for men's health. Testosterone helps build muscle, burn sugar, and reduce inflammation. These three actions have significant implications for what happens to men as their testosterone levels fall. Numerous studies have shown a definite link between low testosterone and an increased risk of heart disease, including heart attacks and congestive heart failure. Testosterone not only helps the heart function better (because the heart is, after all, a big muscle), it actually dilates the arteries that supply blood to the heart and reduces cholesterol plaque formation in the carotid arteries that supply the brain. Men with heart disease who were given testosterone had better performance on stress tests, meaning they could exercise longer without having angina (heart pain). In young men with premature heart disease, testosterone levels were found to be significantly lower than their healthy counterparts. Testosterone also improves blood flow to the brain, leading to better performance on tests of memory, ability to make decisions, and a lower risk for Alzheimer's disease.

Testosterone is a man's most potent anti-inflammatory. This fact is of great importance when we remember that most diseases today are due to inflammation. This includes not only heart disease, as was discussed above, but also diabetes, hypertension, cancer, autoimmune diseases, and even plain old muscle and joint aches.

🍃 Patient Story

Frank, a sixty-four-year-old African-American male, had a heart attack in 1984. He was sent home from the emergency department with no follow-up. Because Frank is a chemist, he began to explore the biochemical response of the body and had come up with a supplement regimen that was helping his angina, but he still had it. On his salivary testing, Frank was both adrenal-fatigued and low in testosterone. I supported his adrenals as well as starting testosterone, and Frank's angina continued to improve.

Why Are Men So Low In Testosterone?

In my practice, I routinely see men in their forties who are low in testosterone. I even have a few twenty-year-olds that are low in testosterone! Why? It is well-documented that testosterone levels around the world have been falling each decade since the 1950s. The biggest reason is toxins in our environment that act like estrogen in the body and reduce the ability of the testicles to function properly. These toxins, called xenoestrogens, are contained in pesticides, solvents and plastics. Xenoestrogens are impossible to avoid.

Another group of toxins that reduce testicular function are heavy metals. (Refer to the adrenal chapter for more information on where we get these toxins.) All heavy metals affect the healthy functioning of the endocrine organs—not just the testicles, but the adrenal glands and the pituitary gland as well.

Speaking of adrenals, stress is another big reason why men have low testosterone. (Again, please refer to the adrenal chapter for a complete discussion on adrenal concerns.) Suffice to say that with increased stress, our bodies go into survival mode. This means that the body shifts reserves from reproduction (something done only when food was plentiful), to surviving a hostile environment. The body will actually steal testosterone to make more cortisol, our primary stress hormone.

Wait a Minute – You're Telling Me Testosterone Will Keep Me Healthy? I Thought it Caused Prostate Cancer!

The myth that testosterone causes prostate cancer has finally been debunked by a well-known urologist from Harvard; Dr. Abraham Morgenteler. Thankfully, he has written several articles and a wonderful book called *Testosterone for Life*, outlining why we should have never bought into this myth in the first place. It all started in the 1940s, with one study of 20 men who had prostate cancer. Drs. Huggins and Hodges castrated men with advanced prostate cancer and found that in several of the cases the patient's metastases started to shrink. They then gave testosterone back to these men who had no testosterone production of their own. In just one patient, the cancer began to grow again. Can you believe it? .For over sixty years now, doctors have believed that testosterone replacement would cause prostate cancer based on ONE patient who already had cancer to begin with!

Dr. Morgenteler has reviewed all of the subsequent studies related to prostate cancer and testosterone replacement and has concluded that there is no relationship whatsoever between serum testosterone levels and prostate cancer risk in longitudinal studies, and no increase in prostate cancer rates in clinical trials of supplemental testosterone.

How did he resolve the findings in the Huggins and Hodges patient? His conclusion is this: a case of "saturation" of the prostate. If a man is low in testosterone and we give him replacement testosterone, the prostate cells, which thrive on testosterone take up the testosterone and become very healthy. Since prostate cancer cells are also prostate cells gone awry, if there are prostate cancer cells already present but microscopic, they will become healthier and seem to grow. So supplemental testosterone can "bring to light" an existing prostate cancer, but does not cause prostate cancer. We can follow this in blood work with a PSA (prostate-specific antigen) blood test. This is the screening test for prostate cancer, and it is often observed that there is an initial increase in the PSA when testosterone is administered, then a gradual decline as the prostate cells become more robust initially. It is important to ensure that the initial increase does not continue— that could indicate that there may be a hidden prostate cancer.

I Went To My Doctor and He Says My Testosterone Level Is Normal

This is where doctors trained in anti-aging medicine differ from traditionally trained medical doctors. We are looking at what levels achieve optimal health, and since it is known that testosterone is key to helping prevent so many illnesses, doctors trained in anti-aging medicine typically want levels to be closer to the levels you had in your thirties, not what might be "normal" for an un-replaced eighty-year-old. Another issue is that traditionally trained doctors look at total levels of testosterone in blood, but the free testosterone level is what needs to be evaluated. In blood, hormones can come three different ways. They can be floating around free and unattached, and are then able to be taken up by the cells and used—this is the part we want to know about, because we are only as healthy as our cells are. The other portions of hormones in blood are either bound to a protein we all make called albumin, or to another protein called sex hormone binding globulin (SHBG). SHBG actually increases with age, so the free portion of the hormone decreases. This means that even if the total testosterone level is adequate, if SHBG is elevated, there could be very little testosterone going into the cells.

🍃 Patient Story

Don, a 43-year-old chiropractor, presented complaining of feeling exhausted and irritable. He was an avid reader and had learned that low testosterone could be the cause of his symptoms, but when his traditionally trained physician had tested his levels, the results were "normal." On further testing I found the free portion of testosterone, the part available for his cells to use, was quite low. With adrenal support and replacement testosterone, he is feeling much better. His energy and mood are improved, and he is able to enjoy life again.

Okay, You Have Convinced Me! How Do I Replace My Testosterone?

Production of testosterone can be increased through things like detoxing heavy metals, eating a diet high in protein, and exercising.

Diet and Nutrition: As we discussed in the adrenal chapter, eating plenty of fresh fruits and vegetables is important to hormone balancing. Avoiding processed foods which are nutrient-deficient and getting enough protein are also very helpful for hormone balancing. For men, the goal is to increase our protein consumption to two grams per kilogram of body weight of protein per day to help the body produce healthy amounts of hormones. This is because men have more muscle mass and, as such, need more protein to both build that muscle and make healthy hormones.

Getting Enough Rest: Remember, this is about balance!.Stress uses up our hormones and turns sex hormones into cortisol for survival. We absolutely have to work on adrenal issues to attempt to balance hormones. This includes getting adequate sleep, having "play" time, and detoxifying heavy metals!

Exercise: Exercise has actually been shown to help with hormone balance because it decreases the amount of testosterone that is converted to estrogen. Men need a little estrogen, but not very much. While exercising decreases the amount of testosterone converting to estrogen, two important things increase estrogen production in men: belly fat and alcohol. Exercise also helps adrenal issues, which significantly helps hormone balancing. It also helps build muscle mass, and muscles make testosterone as well. Exercising is one of the biggest things men can do to increase testosterone production.

Supplements: Those B vitamins are essential! A good B-100 complex is a great place to start, but it is important to add extra B12, as most B complexes do not include enough B12. Also, replacing electrolytes with an electrolyte drink (watch the sugar!), sea salt in water, or alfalfa is crucial to healthy body function and hormone balance. Omega-3 fatty acids help to balance hormones, because healthy fats are needed for hormone production. Zinc is a mineral that is especially important for men, as it decreases that conversion of testosterone to estrogen, and increases prostate health and helps the adrenals. Finally, increasing amino acid intake can help increase testosterone levels. Amino acids are the protein building blocks that make up hormones like testosterone, so ensuring the body has enough on board is helpful. A good quality branched-chain amino acid complex can be taken daily.

Patient Story

John, a forty-six-year-old self-proclaimed "gym rat," works out for an hour and a half every day. He was recently diagnosed with low testosterone by his primary care physician, who then referred him to an endocrinologist. The endocrinologist wanted to start him on replacement therapy, but John wanted to know why he was low in testosterone. After his work-up, he was found to be heavy metal toxic and needed to improve his protein intake. While I started testosterone replacement early on, we have been able to cut back on his dose now that he is no longer heavy metal toxic.

Beyond The Basics – Testosterone Replacement

If all of the outlined efforts are not enough to achieve adequate levels, testosterone replacement is in order. It is very important to use bio-identical testosterone. The term bio-identical means that it is made to be the exact same molecule your body makes, whereas testosterone made by pharmaceutical companies is different than what your body would naturally make. Testosterone comes in creams, injections or little pills called troches (troh-kees) that you can dissolve under your tongue.

I never, ever use oral testosterone, because it has been shown to increase inflammation in the liver. If the dose is high enough, it can actually cause liver cancer. The method that is best for you is an individual preference. Injections should be given weekly to minimize the peaks and valleys in dosing that come with weekly use. Creams and troches are used once daily. With these forms following your testosterone levels is a little more challenging, because creams and troches do not reliably show up in blood. They are best followed with saliva testing and monitoring of symptoms. Injectable testosterone can be given in the thigh once weekly. While blood levels of injectable testosterone can be reliably followed, there are problems of peaks and troughs. Basically, your testosterone levels will be higher shortly after the injection and lower just before the injection.

Use of supplemental testosterone can have a few side effects. The blood can thicken in men on testosterone, which may cause an increase in clotting. This can be followed through blood testing. When men are on too much testosterone, they can also experience testicular shrinkage, joint pain, and irritability. It is interesting how the symptoms of too little testosterone are similar to the symptoms of too much!

In Summary

I hope I have convinced you that optimal testosterone levels in men are a big part of maintaining a healthy, active lifestyle and preventing disease – not just having fun in bed!

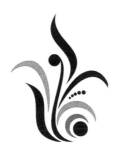

Chapter 4

Why am I so tired?
Is my thyroid off?

Why Am I So Tired?
Is My Thyroid Off?

Do you feel tired all the time? Do you have mental fog? Do you feel blah, like you just don't enjoy life? Are you constipated? Are you sensitive to temperature extremes? Is your hair falling out? You could have thyroid disease!

What is the Thyroid?

The thyroid is a gland that sits at the base of our neck and is responsible for controlling the metabolic rate of our entire bodies. Our active thyroid hormone (T3) controls how fast cells work, how much work cells do, and how many molecules of energy cells produce. Without an optimally working thyroid gland, we feel sluggish, we may have trouble losing weight, or our thought processes may become more difficult. In essence, we have "slowed down."

🍃 Patient Story

When Shelley went through menopause, her entire outlook on life changed. While she had been active and stress-free, she was now more depressed and had much less energy. Shelley had done her homework—she knew replacement hormones would be helpful, and they were to a point. However, when we finally added thyroid hormone, Shelley felt like the sun came out. Her mood improved, her energy improved, and she felt back to her old self.

How Does The Thyroid Work?

As with all glands and hormones, the thyroid gland is a finely tuned organ that responds to feedback mechanisms from throughout the body. This is how it works: The pituitary gland in the brain produces thyroid-stimulating hormone (TSH). This travels through the blood to stimulate the thyroid to produce thyroxine (T4). T4 is a protein with four iodine molecules attached to it. It is not the active form of thyroid hormone. T4 needs to be taken up by the cells in the body and have an iodine molecule cleaved off, converting it to T3. The conversion of T4 to T3 takes zinc, selenium, and iodine, so if these minerals are low, this conversion will not be adequate. T3 is then the active form of thyroid hormone that travels through the body, stimulating the metabolic rate of all of our cells. T4 also travels back to the brain, informing our pituitary glands about how much is being produced. This feedback loop is then what tells our pituitary gland how much TSH should be produced. Here is the interesting twist: T4 can also be converted to a molecule called reverse T3. Reverse T3 is the mirror image of T3 and, as such, can bind to the T3 receptor sites. Instead of producing stimulation, reverse T3 just sits there and does nothing. It actually prevents T3 from binding, so reverse T3 makes the entire metabolism slower. If there is a lot of reverse T3, even if the other numbers look good, you will still feel hypothyroid (slow thyroid). Reverse T3 production is stimulated by three things: stress, heavy metal toxicity, and an elevated serum insulin level.

🍃 Patient Story

Judy initially came to me for BHRT. However, when I did a complete work-up, it seemed like her adrenals were the bigger issue. She had a very busy life, with many social engagements and two teenage children. Her cortisol was low and reverse T3 was high. Judy's body had the brakes on big time! After what seemed like forever—about a year of detoxing and supporting her adrenals—her reverse T3 finally started coming down.

What Does Thyroid Hormone Do?

Because the thyroid regulates the metabolism of all of our cells, you can imagine that the thyroid is an essential and vital part of the optimal functioning of our bodies. Low levels of active thyroid hormone have been particularly implicated in heart disease, and especially in congestive heart failure. The optimum functioning of our brain cells requires adequate levels of thyroid hormone. When our thyroid is not functioning properly, we suffer brain fog, slow thinking, and depression. Every cell in our gut requires thyroid hormone. Our bodies cannot absorb and digest nutrients without optimal thyroid.

Here is a short list of symptoms of hypothyroidism:

- Fatigue

- Constipation

- Muscle weakness

- Depression

- Weight gain or difficulty losing weight

- Irritability

- Coarse, dry hair

- Memory loss

- Dry, rough skin

- Hair loss

- Heat and cold intolerance

- Decreased libido

- Muscle cramps and frequent aches

- Swelling

- Abnormal menstrual cycles

- Migraines

How Do Thyroid Problems Start?

Our thyroid glands are taking a hit in our 21st century world, for two basic reasons. First of all, most of us experience too much stress. Because of our higher levels of stress, our levels of inflammation are also much higher than in previous generations. As I discussed in the adrenal chapter, stress increases our inflammation. The thyroid also seems to be one of our genetic "weak links," so to speak. Increased inflammation can occur at any point in the body where there is a genetic weak link. When the thyroid is the genetic weak link, the body may produce antibodies against the thyroid. This means that because there is so much inflammation, the body's immune system is on overdrive and it gets confused. The body actually starts attacking the thyroid rather than legitimate invaders like bacteria and viruses. After a while, this, of course, affects thyroid function. The presence of thyroid antibodies can increase a woman's risk for breast cancer by sixty percent in her lifetime.

Another reason why stress affects our thyroid gland is because cortisol, our "fight-or-flight" hormone, affects thyroid metabolism at every level. If our cortisol is too high or too low (adrenaline high vs. adrenal fatigue), all levels of thyroid hormone production are decreased, from production of TSH in the brain to production of T4, to conversion of T4 to T3, while production of reverse T3 increases. This makes sense from an evolutionary standpoint. If we think of when we had prolonged cortisol issues "back in the day," it was often when we were starving through winter, and our bodies were trying to slow down metabolism to ensure our survival into spring.

The second reason why thyroid disease is so prevalent is because of environmental toxins. While many toxins affect the thyroid gland, the biggest problem is bromide. Bromide is a chemical that is used in fabrics as a fire-retardant. Bromide is sprayed into our mattresses, chair cushions, carpets, and even children's clothing. Basically, bromide is everywhere. There is no common testing for bromine because virtually everyone is toxic. Because they are chemically so similar, bromide displaces iodine in the thyroid, so that the thyroid and thyroid hormones do not work as well. Interestingly, chloride does the same thing, so for people who swim a lot or have high exposures to chlorine, thyroid problems are common.

What Thyroid Studies Should I Be Tested For?

Most doctors only test for TSH. The problem with this is that TSH is simply a feedback hormone and does not tell us the actual level of thyroid hormone. TSH reveals nothing about how the body is converting T4 to T3, or how much reverse T3 is being made. A complete thyroid check should include: TSH, free T4, free T3, reverse T3, anti-thyroid peroxidase antibodies and anti-thyroglobulin antibodies. Because cortisol so directly affects the thyroid, it is essential that cortisol levels be checked as well.

Remember that whenever doctors are testing hormones, we either need to get the free portion of the hormone—that part of the hormone in blood that is available to the cell to use, or we need to test through saliva. This is why we want to evaluate free T3 and free T4 in blood, rather than total T3 or total T4. When doctors check the total T3 or T4, they are not getting an accurate picture of what is available to be taken up and used by the cell. A significant part of that total amount could be bound to thyroglobulin, the thyroid hormones carrier protein, and not available to the cell to take up and use.

Another question in checking thyroid studies is: What are optimal levels? Even among traditional doctors, the acceptable level of TSH has changed over the years. In the 1970s, 10 micro international units per milliliter was considered an acceptable TSH level. Currently, Family Physicians and Internists feel a TSH up to 5.5 micro international units per milliliter is normal. Endocrinologists want a TSH to be less than 2.5 micro international units per milliliter, but often will not replace thyroid until the TSH reaches 5.5 micro international units per milliliter Anti-aging doctors understand the importance of an extremely well-functioning thyroid, and look for TSH levels to be less than or equal to 1.5 micro international units per milliliter.

Here are other optimal thyroid hormone levels:

Free T4   1.4-1.8 nanograms per deciliter

Free T3   3.3-4.2 picograms per milliliter

Reverse T3   Less than or equal to 20 nanograms per deciliter

Treating Thyroid Problems

Treating suboptimal thyroid levels can be a complicated process, because cortisol issues first need to be addressed first and foremost. If our state of "fight/flight" is not adequately treated before replacing thyroid hormone, significant problems can occur. For example, if there is adrenal fatigue, it is like we have no gas in the tank. If we then try to use thyroid medicine, it is like pushing our foot down on the accelerator when we have no gas in the tank. Like a car, we just rev our engines, which for bodies can mean heart palpitations.

If you have adrenal problems, a great place to start to support your thyroid would be to replace minerals like zinc and selenium, along with iodine. Zinc can be taken in doses of 30 milligrams per day, and selenium should be around 200 micrograms per day. My favorite form of iodine comes as Iodoral, which is actually a combination of iodine and iodide. The thyroid preferentially takes up the iodide, and other tissues that are dependent on iodine, such as breasts, ovaries, and testicles, will take up the iodine. Iodoral comes in 12.5 milligram tablets and typically one-half tablet, or 6.25 milligrams daily, is adequate.

If you are diagnosed with suboptimal thyroid hormone levels, it is very important to evaluate your reverse T3 level. If it is high, you will need to cleanse for heavy metals and examine the stress in your life. Cleansing for heavy metals often includes using alginates like Chlorella or blue-green algae, which bind heavy metals and pull them out through the intestinal tract. (Please refer to the adrenal chapter for ways to deal with heavy metals and stress.) As mentioned previously, optimal thyroid function also requires minerals like selenium and zinc, along with iodine. Vitamin D levels also affect thyroid, and should be optimized by taking 4000 IU/day for adults.

If your thyroid is still suboptimal, it is much better to replace thyroid hormone with a desiccated pig glandular thyroid, like a medication called Armour Thyroid. Pigs actually have the exact same thyroid hormone as humans, so not only is this a more natural approach, but studies show that people actually feel better on Armour. Armour thyroid is a combination of T4 and T3, whereas most of the pharmaceutical thyroid preparations like Synthroid and Levothyroxine are 100 percent T4. This means that we are completely relying on the body to produce T3, and in some cases this can drive up the production of reverse T3. Some people with thyroid antibodies do not tolerate Armour, and will need to use a combination of synthetic T4 and T3.

Thyroid problems can be complex and are interconnected with all our other hormones, even our sex hormones. Therefore, other than supporting the thyroid nutritionally, I typically do not prescribe thyroid hormone until after working on cortisol and sex hormones for a few months. However, once I get thyroid in place, it is often the last step to get to optimal health!

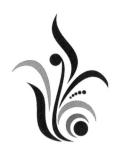

Chapter 5

Conclusion & Recommended Reading

Conclusion

So there you have it. We have traveled through the basics of hormone health—but not just hormone health, as hormone health is the foundation of total health—first with the adrenals and cortisol issues, where we learned how the stresses of our lives affect our well-being. Next we moved on to the sex hormones, which are essential to the healthy functioning of every cell in our bodies, and how our cells communicate with each other. And finally, we explored our butterfly-shaped thyroid gland, which affects the rate at which our cells function. The thyroid can be the icing on the cake of our optimal health when we fine-tune its balance. These three critical areas provide the foundation of our physical health.

Every day I see patients in my office who have been suffering from poor health and feel stuck in it. They walk through their lives feeling less than optimal, being tired, cranky, or just feeling badly. Sometimes we get so used to feeling poorly that we forget what it is to feel great. I firmly believe that an important part of my role as a physician is to hold the "space of wellness" for my patients. Even if my patients do not remember what it is like to feel optimal, it is my job as their physician to remember for them.

I hope this book will help you on the path toward your optimal health and healing. Our goal in this lifetime is, after all, to become the very best version of ourselves that we can be. Sometimes good health can feel like a moving target, but the times we achieve feeling great are so wonderful that we are encouraged and challenged to feel fantastic all of the time. We are like onions—always peeling back the layers toward health and wholeness. Health is never a straight and narrow path. We may peel back a layer of some issues that have been bothering us, only to discover a deeper issue that needs to be worked on. However, as we work through these layers, we can often be astounded at how great we can feel. The only limitation on our optimal health is what we believe our optimal health can be!

Recommended Reading

LaValle, James, RPh., CCN., ND. *Cracking the Metabolic Code: 9 Keys to Optimal Health.* Laguna Beach, CA. Basic Health Publications, Inc. 2004.

Wilson, James, ND., DC., PhD. *Adrenal Fatigue: The 21st Century Stress Syndrome.* Petaluma, CA. Smart Publications. 2001.

Smith, Pamela, MD, MPH. *What You Must Know About Women's Hormones. Your Guide to Natural Hormone Treatments for PMS, Menopause, Osteoporosis, PCOS, and More.* Garden City Park, New York. Square One Publishers.

Lee, John, MD and Hanley, Jesse, MD. *What Your Doctor May NOT Tell You About Pre-menopause.* Grand Central Publishing. New York, New York.

Brownstein, David, MD. *Iodine: Why You Need it, Why You Can't Live without It.* Medical Alternatives Press. West Bloomfield, MI. Print. 2002.

Mortengaler, Abraham, MD. *Testosterone for Life.* United States. Harvard University and McGraw Hill. Print. 2009.

Brownstein, David, MD. *Overcoming Thyroid Disorders.* Medical Alternatives Press. West Bloomfield, MI. 2002. Print.

D'Adamo, Peter, ND. *Eat Right 4 Your Type. The IndividuaLillyed Diet Solution to Staying Healthy, Living Longer & Achieving Your Ideal Weight.* G.P. Putnam's Sons. New York, New York. Print. 1996.

Glossary of Terms

ATP: a phosphorylated nucleotide C10H16N5O13P3, composed of adenosine and three phosphate groups, that supplies energy for many biochemical cellular processes by undergoing enzymatic hydrolysis, especially to ADP—called also adenosine triphosphate

ACTH hormone: a protein hormone of the anterior lobe of the pituitary gland that stimulates the adrenal cortex—called also adrenocorticotropic hormone

Adrenal fatigue: a collection of signs and symptoms resulting from poor functioning of the adrenal glands

Adrenal gland: either of a pair of complex endocrine organs near the anterior medial border of the kidney, consisting of a mesodermal cortex that produces glucocorticoid, mineralocorticoid, androgenic hormones and an ectodermal medulla that produces epinephrine and norepinephrine—called also adrenal, suprarenal gland

Albumin: any of numerous simple heat-coagulable, water-soluble proteins that occur in blood plasma or serum, muscle, the whites of eggs, milk, and other animal substances and in many plant tissues and fluids

Aldosterone: a steroid hormone $C_{21}H_{28}O_5$ of the adrenal cortex that functions in the regulation of the salt and water balance of the body

Autoimmune: of, relating to, or caused by autoantibodies or T cells that attack molecules, cells, or tissues of the organism producing them <autoimmune diseases.

Cardiovascular: of, relating to, or involving the heart and blood vessels

Cortisol: a glucocorticoid $C_{21}H_{30}O_5$ produced by the adrenal cortex upon stimulation by ACTH that mediates various metabolic processes (as gluconeogenesis), has anti-inflammatory and immunosuppressive properties, and whose levels in the blood may become elevated in response to physical or psychological stress —called also hydrocortisone

DHEA: dehydroepiandrosterone: a weakly androgenic ketosteroid C19H28O2 secreted by the adrenal glands that is an intermediate in the biosynthesis of testosterone and estrogens (as estradiol); also : a synthetic derivative of this compound—abbr DHEA

Electrolytes: any of the ions (as of sodium or calcium) that in biological fluid regulate or affect most metabolic processes (as the flow of nutrients into and waste products out of cells)

Epinephrine: a colorless crystalline, feebly basic sympathomimetic hormone C9H13NO3 that is the principal blood-pressure-raising hormone secreted by the adrenal medulla and is used medicinally, especially as a heart stimulant, a vasoconstrictor in controlling hemorrhages of the skin, and a muscle relaxant in bronchial asthma—called also adrenaline

Estrogen: any of various natural steroids (as estradiol) that are formed from androgen precursors, that are secreted chiefly by the ovaries, placenta, adipose tissue, and testes, and that stimulate the development of female secondary sex characteristics and promote the growth and maintenance of the female reproductive system

Heavy metals: metals that have a molecular weight greater than that of water. Metals that are in higher amounts than should naturally occur due to industrialization

Hormone: a product of living cells that circulates in body fluids (as blood) or sap and produces a specific often stimulatory effect on the activity of cells usually remote from its point of origin; also : a synthetic substance that acts like a hormone

Immune System: the bodily system that protects the body from foreign substances, cells, and tissues by producing the immune response and that includes especially the thymus, spleen, lymph nodes, special deposits of lymphoid tissue (as in the gastrointestinal tract and bone marrow), macrophages, lymphocytes including the B cells and T cells, and antibodies

Natural Killer Cell: a large granular lymphocyte capable of killing a tumor or microbial cell without prior exposure to the target cell and without having it presented with or marked by a histocompatibility antigen—called also NK cell

Neurotransmitters: a substance (as norepinephrine or acetylcholine) that transmits nerve impulses across a synapse

Norepinephrine: a monoamine C8H11NO3: is a eurotransmitter in postganglionic neurons of the sympathetic nervous system and in some parts of the central nervous system, is a vasopressor hormone of the adrenal medulla, and is a precursor of epinephrine in its major biosynthetic pathway

Ovary: one of the typically paired essential female reproductive organs that produce eggs, and in vertebrates female sex hormones

Pituitary Gland: a small oval endocrine organ that is attached to the infundibulum of the brain, consists of an epithelial anterior lobe joined by an intermediate part to a posterior lobe of nervous origin, and produces various internal secretions directly or indirectly impinging on most basic body functions —called also hypophysis, pituitary body

Progesterone: a female steroid sex hormone C21H30O2 that is secreted by the corpus luteum to prepare the endometrium for implantation and later by the placenta during pregnancy to prevent rejection of the developing embryo or fetus; also : a synthetic steroid resembling progesterone in action

Are you tired all the time? Worn out?

Do you feel like you are not enjoying your

life as much as you want to?

Or perhaps you feel moody and irritable, and

you snap at your loved ones?

In her latest book, *Hormone Balancing: the Basics*, Dr. Leila Kirdani reveals how stress can affect our energy levels and cause our sex-hormones and thyroid to be out of balance. Hormones are essential messengers between cells and help to keep us healthy and functioning well. Learn how you can overcome the effects of stress and feel wonderful!

About Dr. Leila Kirdani

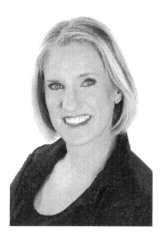

Dr. Leila Kirdani began her medical journey as a traditional Family Physician, practicing in both rural and urban areas of the country. Over time she saw more clearly that what traditional medicine has to offer is limited and does not truly address the underlying causes of bodily dysfunction.

She went on to complete a fellowship in anti-aging, regenerative, and functional medicine which has allowed her to combine her love of natural medicine with her more traditional medical background. Dr. Kirdani has been helping patients achieve an excellent quality of life for over five years in her home town of Rochester, New York.

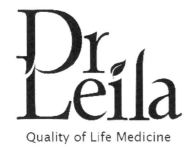

Quality of Life Medicine

4414 Culver Road
Rochester NY 14622
(585) 773-4777
www.drleila.com

For additional copies go to Amazon.com or anywhere books are sold.

For Multiple or Educational discounts go to www.DrLeila.com

For Keynote Speaker go to Dr.Leila Kirdani

email drleilak@gmail.com

For Appointment call the office

More from Dr Leila

Check for it Everywhere

GET THE
SKINNY HCG

Human Chorionic Gonadotropin

How to achieve
your optimum weight
and improve your
health with HCG

Leila Kirdani, M.D.

Notes

Notes

Notes

Notes

Notes

Notes

Made in the USA
Charleston, SC
25 January 2014